# On Fi:

# Radical Cure
## by Medicines

*by*
**J. Compton Burnett, M.D.**

*Reprinted from the*
**Second Revised & Enlarged Edition**

*"Men will not heed! Yet were I not prepared*
*With better refuge for them, tongue of mine*
*Should ne'er reveal how blank their dwelling is;*
*I would sit down in silence with the. rest".*
—Browning's "Paracelsus"

**B. Jain Publishers (P) Ltd.**
USA—EUROPE—INDIA

**ON FISTULA AND ITS RADICAL CURE BY MEDICINES**

Second Revised & Enlarged Edition
10th Impression: 2016

**Note From the Publishers**

This book is a part of special "Low Price Editions" series, which has specially been made for students and has books at prices you would love.

Published by Kuldeep Jain for
**B. JAIN PUBLISHERS (P) LTD.**
B. Jain House, D-157, Sector-63,
NOIDA-201307, U.P. (INDIA)
Tel.: +91-120-4933333 • Email: info@bjain.com
Website: **www.bjain.com**

Printed in India
B B Press  Noida
ISBN: 978-81-319-0785-6

# PREFACE

During the past fifteen years a considerable number of cases of diseases of the anal and intercrural regions have been under my professional care, notably cases of haemorrhoids and varicocele; and intercurrently with these not a few cases of fistula have come under my observation. At first I did not quite believe it possible to cure fistula with medicines alone without any operation or topical applications, for I had been taught that to cure a fistula you must need to operate upon it. So you will not find anything about fistula in works on Medicine. I pulled down a dozen master works at random from my shelves, Kafka, Grauvogl, Kissel, Guttceit, Rademacher, and the like and found either nothing at all, or passing reference to fistula merely. Fistula belongs to the surgeons. But I had also been taught that piles cannot be cured without operation and as I found this teaching false and untrue (having myself cured numbers of such cases with homoeopathic treatment alone). I set about the treatment of fistula also with medicines, and frequently succeeded in my task, mostly with the help of the experience of eminent homoeopathic physicians, whose written testimony any inquirer may find for himself on reference to the literature of the homoeopathic school. With the lapse of time my own experience has grown, and I have found that not only haemorrhoids, but also fistula can be genuinely and radically cured with medicines alone, a knowledge of homoeopathy, a little patience, and diagnostic skill being given.

It is unfortunate for the progress and extension of Scientific Medicines, and by Scientific Medicine I mean no more and no less; than Homoeopathy it is unfortunate, I say, that our surgeons are so clever with their hands, for they do their work for the most part so well, so neatly, so painlessly, that medical men have come to rely more and more upon the knife, to the almost total exclusion of the more gentle, more humane, and more rational treatment with medicines.

The medical profession at large condemn homoeopathy, they know nothing about it. There was a time when I also condemned it, I also then knew nothing about it but now, having studied it and practised it, my contempt has given place to humble-minded thankfulness and I maintain that homoeopathy, real scientific homoeopathy, is the most mighty weapon against any disease known to mankind. It is in the hope that other may share this knowledge that I send these pages to the press.

2, Finsbury Circus, E. C.      **J. COMPTON BURNETT**

March, 1894.

# CONTENTS

# PART II

# PART I

There are various kinds of cure in practical medical life; given a case of fistula that is treated by applying healing remedies to the same, it may thus be brought to heal up. This healing up is commonly designated as cure. In the sense of *curare*, this is, of course, correct; but I hardly think it is so in the true meaning of our English word to *cure*. But to obviate any misapprehension, I mean in this little treatise by cure a radical proceeding aimed at the constitutional cause or root of the complaint, and not a forcible healing up, by medicines applied to the suffering part. The word fistula means in Latin a *pipe*, such as a water-pipe or wind-pipe. In medical language it signifies a really or assumedly pipe-shaped canal in the living tissue, and may occur in various regions of the body. We are here principally concerned with fistula as it is found near the anus-*fistula-in-ano*, one case only, and that a very remarkable one of urinary fistula being narrated.* In common medicochirurgical practice, it is held and taught that the fistular canal cannot heal, either because the fistula being internal (complete or incomplete) flatus and faecal matter constantly irritate it, and thus prevent the healing process or else because of the lining of the fistula itself becoming a secreting membrane-pyogenic or otherwise. Hence it is useful to slit open the fistula, and thus turn it into a wound, which is then cleansed and dressed with some antiseptic or vulnerary, to the end that the same may heal up. At first sight this seems the only rational mode of treating fistula, so that the individual may not be debilitated by the discharge and local misery.

It has, however, long been contended by able medical thinkers that the fistular process is the local expression of a constitutional cause, and that the true philosophical and scientific way of treating fistula is to remove the said constitutional cause, and then the fistula will heal of itself with little or no local aid at all.

---

*In the Second Part, however, other cases are now added-AUTHOR.

We will call these two theories respectively that of the *localist* and that of the *constitutionalists*.

I take the stand of those who hold that fistula is most commonly a constitutional affection, and must therefore be treated by the physician. I go further and maintain that the local treatment of dyscratic fistula is not only wrong, but irrational and harmful. In many cases it is better to leave such a fistula alone than cause it to heal by operation and antiseptic (or other) dressings. Theories to be of any service must be workable in practice. The localists-the surgeons operate upon their fistula patients, and publish their results. I treat my fistula patients with medicines, and here given some results. Let these respective results be compared. But this comparison of results should take into account the *future* life and health history of the patient. On this part of the question hinges the whole thing. I do not deny that fistula can often be successfully operated upon and made to close up, but what of the future health of the individual? There's the rub.

But whatever view may be held of the true nature of fistula (using the word as commonly employed), I shall in the following pages prove that fistula can be radically cured by medicines, and that is all I claim for merit of these pages. Incidentally the remedies found useful are given, so that the competent may judge for themselves, and the inexperienced learn how to do it if they so elect. The key to the use of the remedies is the law of similars; the guide to their choice, the patient's symptoms, subjective and objective.

As before remarked, fistula in the anal region and piles are not, always duly differentiated from one another by the sufferers, and hence it happens that those practitioners who see a good deal of one complaint are pretty sure to see a good deal of the other. Myself, I have had a rather wide experience in the medicinal treatment of haemorrhoids*, and intercurrently a certain number of fistula have passed under my observation and professional care, and from the experience thus acquired, I can say that fistula-in-ano may usually be completely cured by medicines. And I think that there can hardly be any two opinions as to the superiority of the cure of fistula by remedies over its operative treatment. I say operative treatment, for in operative cure I do not indeed believe; you may slit open a fistula and cause it to heal up, but the fistular patient is constitutionally precisely where he was before. That surely every thoughtful person, whether patient or physician, or even surgeon,

---

*See my "Diseases of the Veins"

must concede. There are, no doubt, certain cases of fistula in which we are obliged to have recourse to the knife or other surgical operation, but I am firmly convinced this need not often be the case, indeed, hardly ever, provided the right medicinal treatment be begun early enough and persevered in long enough. Even those whose only means of treating fistula is surgery have, nevertheless, to admit their utter and absolute powerlessness in a very large number of cases of this most distressing complaint, and, unfortunately for the poor sufferers, the cases in which the surgeons dare not operate, on account of contingent poitrinary explosions or exacerbations, or because the fistulae will not heal, even though they were operated upon, just these very cases are the worst and most serious. In fact, in really dyscratic cases of fistula, the surgeon's knife is of no more use than the north wind. And, indeed, how should it be possible for local work to cure a constitutional ailment, which fistula undoubtedly is nine times out of every ten? It is not possible. The diathesis must be mended and then the fistula heals, and after certain flickerings comes no more; the patient gets a healthier colour and takes on flesh, and with it comes health and strength. Of course, I do not advocate the medicinal treatment of traumatic fistula from fish bones imbeded in passing down athwart the gut, lacerating it, and then the faeces irritate, set up inflammation, which together burrow into the tissues, form sinuses and fistulae; nor do I advocate leaving bags of scrofulous pus pent up; not at all, here let surgery step in, and that promptly. But these cases are not the most common by any means nor would I for one moment be understood to deny that the poor person suffering from fistula, living under unhygienic conditions, ill-fed, and badly cared for, I say I would not for an instant be understood to say that such patients are not much improved, and perhaps even cured, when brought into a nice clean hospital, well-fed, dosed with cod-liver-oil and tonics, and their fistulae operated upon.

Common sense and actual facts forbid. I am thinking of the clean living, well-fed sufferers from fistula, who still suffer notwithstanding easy circumstances, faultless hygiene, and every attention to their physical well being. These are the cases I am familiar with, and of these I write. I will now close in a little upon my task, and proceed to show the way in which anal fistula may be medicinally treated without any operation or local messing and pottering at all, and not only medicinally *treated*, but also medicinally radically *cured*. The following series of detailed cases will also prove that the right remedies will help where surgery has failed, for the very best surgical treatment fails much more frequently than surgeons, I know of, are willing to confess. Not that I impute bad faith to them, but it takes a good deal to convince even the most honest against their will. I think I could hardly do better than begin with a case of recurrent fistula, because it seems to me that if a complaint recur over and over again at any given spot, there must need be an internal cause for such recurrence; if not, whence does the prefistular abscess come?

## RECURRENT CIRCUMANAL ABSCESS AND FISTULA

On May 22, 1882, a married London merchant, thirty seven years of age, called to consult me in regard to recurrent fistula and circumanal abscess. He related to me that eighteen months previously he got an abscess at the seat, which his surgeon lanced and treated, and in the end pronounced as cured. Cured it was, in the surgeon's opinion; he was quite honest in this expressed opinion, but you might as well say that when you have plucked the apples from your apple trees in the autumn, you have cured the said apple trees of apple bearing, for, although the surgeon had '*cured*' the abscess he had not cured the patient of his power to produce more fistula leading abscesses, in as much as the disease had returned each subsequent spring and fall. And this is really the point I am contending for, viz. the abscess at the seat with its sequential fistula is not disease in its real essence, but only its local expression in the anal region. Not being satisfied with his '*cure*', patient had consulted other surgeons, in all three, for his anal trouble, and all three alike lanced and poulticed, and still it came afresh. On examination I found he was suffering from an incomplete internal fistula that had also just been diagnosed by a noted specialist for diseases of the rectum who had lately seen it, and urged the imperative necessity of cutting it at once.

Patient had a good deal of acne on his shoulders and neck, the eruption often showing white, mattery heads. He had only been vaccinated once, and that as a baby, has had often and many little indolent boils in the nape.

R

*Kalium carbonicum* 30.

June 12–He is much better, the opening of the fistula is now about the size of a split pea.

℞

*Psorinum* 30 in very infrequent doses.

*July* 16–He is not so comfortable at the anus, and the fistula seems more active.

℞

*Thuja occidentalis* 30 in very infrequent doses.

*September* 19–There is great improvement in the anal trouble, and the skin of his neck and shoulders and nape is much healthier and clearer.

℞

*Mercurius corrosivus* in the same strength as *Kalium carbonicum, Psorinum* and *Thuja occidentalis.*

*Jan.* 15, 1883–Fistula well, but there are still blind boils in his skin.

℞

*Aqua silicata*, which finished the cure.

But in the autumn of 1883 another abscess formed, when the same kind of treatment, together with *Arctium lappa; Calcarea carbonica.* etc., was helpful and finally in the spring of 1884, patient paid me three visits with what might be called the last faint flickerings of his fistula disease. Since then ten years have elapsed, and there has been no return, and no attempt at a return, and patient continues otherwise in excellent health. This I know, because he lately brought his wife to me for another matter relating to her health, when I gathered the fact just narrated.

From the circumstances that the disease in this gentleman was some little time before it was quite extinguished, and from the nature of the remedies which acted best and from a certain number of other similar and dissimilar cases, I am quite satisfied that there is fistula and fistula, that it must, in fact, be looked upon as a generic term for several constitutional complaints of a totally different nature, and that surgery of all and every kind is absolutely inadequate to cope with these various constitutional states grouped together under the conventional term fistula. I think the good result obtained by the aid of the knife are partly due to more attention to diet and hygiene and partly to the fact that the fistulous processes themselves may be helped to heal up by antiseptics and cleansing washes. But we must ever bear in mind that forcibly healing a fistula does not necessarily restore the fistula patient to health.  ·

When speak of *health* I do not necessarily mean that every patient with fistula feels ill, for such is not the case, in as much as we meet with quite a number of patients with fistula who can hardly be said to be subjectively ill at all, and yet we could hardly maintain that a man or woman with acne, blind boils, and fistula is in good health. The reason why they do not feel ill lies probably in the fact that these external expressions of ill-health carry out from the blood and internal parts, the *materis morbi* and their being successfully landed on to the outer surface, the internal feeling of well-being is not disturbed. Still, you will generally notice that persons with fistula have a more or less unhealthy skin, which is cheesy, greasy, spotty, pimply, or dirty looking, and they are also commonly anaemic.

Thus the gentleman whose case I have just narrated, when he came to me felt fairly well, but he looked pasty and pale, and his flesh was flabby, now he not only feels well but looks it, and I have no doubt whatever that his future life is now much more safe, and I think it would be only fair if his life insurance company were to pay the fees he incurred.

## SIMPLE FISTULA

The most simple form, however, in which fistula comes before one is where the subjects are seemingly in good health, and in whom the whole thing can be cured by medicines in two or three months. Thus a gentleman of some forty-six years of age, hale and hearty to all appearance consulted me for fistula-in-ano that had plagued him for a number of months. An operation had been decided upon, and assented to by the gentleman, but as he was not exactly ill, and was, moreover, over head and ears in big affairs, he constantly put it off.

It never occurred to him even that medicines were any good in such cases; his own surgeon said they were not and that was enough. The foul discharge was the only thing that really inconvenienced him, with a certain amount or local irritation, and a little blood once in a while but it did not heal, and one day he met with a gentleman, an old friend of his own, and whom I had cured of severe fistula several years previously; the result was that he came to me. Under *Hydrastis canadensis* he got quite well in a little less than two months. No local application of any kind was used. He was more pleased at his rapid cure as he was about to marry at the time, and a fistula is not desirable under such circumstances.

I am in a little doubt as to the origin of the primary morbid element in the case. It was certainly not constitutional to him and 1 am inclined to think it was a local affair acquired *in der wilden Ehe*, and in this particular case, no doubt, an operation with antiseptic dressings would have cured him quite as well as my treatment, though not so pleasantly. Surgeons seem to think there is a kind of spartan virtue in having one's fistula operated upon. I cannot quite see it in that light myself.

## HEPATIC FISTULA

I may not, perhaps, be justified in designating the kind of fistula I here refer to as *hepatic*, but at any rate one meets with certain people with fistula that have enlarged livers as concomitants, and our common hepatics readily cure them. *Chelidonium majus*, *Carduus marianus*, *Myrica cerifera* and *Berberis vulgaris* (as the case may be), cure the liver and at the same time the fistula. They are simple and probably either not constitutional at all, or only in a very slight degree and they do not readily recur. I do not regard them as particularly important, and therefore will not dwell upon them. I have sometimes thought they may be due to high living and want of exercise. There may also be a slight strumous taint at the bottom of them.

## CIRCUMANAL ABSCESS

This is the common origin of fistula, and its treatment is

highly important. I so rarely use local applications at all in any complaints that I will pause here, and, under the heading of circumanal abscess, I will say that the very best plan (where the pain and distress are very great) is to keep the gathering constantly moistened with rag dipped in *Liquor calcis*, P. B. changing the rags very frequently. I shall not easily forget a gentleman I once attended for perennial abscess, in which the pains were extremely severe. Troubles about the anus are, in my experience, for the most part distressing ones, even if only slight. Well, this gentleman, in my judgment, was ridding his organism of a tuberculous tendency by means of this perennial abscess i.e. the organism was brimming over at the part to save the lungs, so I was particularly anxious not to have the abscess interfered with, for I have noticed that cutting open immature abscesses is no gain, they simply go on 'sweating', for double the time it would have taken to heal had the abscesses been allowed to mature in their own way. But he really could not bear the pain; when I applied lime-water rags, with the result that the pain became a mere nothing, and patient forthwith had a beautiful sleep. He made a capital recovery, and fistula was prevented. The principal remedies used were *Aconitum napellus, Silicea terra, Hepar sulphur, Calcarea sulphuricum* and *China officinalis*; with one or two subsequently given constitutional remedies, foremost being *Kalium carbonicum* 30 and *Lappa major* θ.

For the relief of the pain of acute gatherings I have very great confidence in limewater rags. I have often felt very thankful to this excellent practical tip that I first learned of Dr. George Wyld, of London, and if my reading memory does not deceive me, it was a favourite little clinical knack of no less a man than Theophrastus Von Hohenheim, commonly called Paracelsus, and a splendid friend in need it is. I once had a case of gastritis near Hyde Park that resisted all my remedies, and began to look very ugly indeed, when I applied abdominal compresses saturated with *Liquor calcis*, P. B. and frequently changed, patient had a good sleep within two hours, and returned home to her friends in the country within a week.

In advocating the medicinal treatment of fistula (which I should certainly prefer to call the *Fistular Disease*), I am stepping out of the serried ranks of the profession to some extent, and am therefore by no means medically catholic or orthodox. Still there are others who have done, and do the same thing. I mention this lest I be understood to give out that I have myself originated the cure of anal fistula by medicines. This is not so.

## PHYSICIANS WHO TREAT FISTULA MEDICINALLY

Before proceeding any further, I will quote the doings and sayings of a number of physicians more or less like-minded with myself.

Thus:

Dr. Kidd ('Laws of Therapeutics', p-174) shows that whether we profess homoeopathy or not, we require its teachings to cure our patients. He says: 'Fistula-in-ano cured by dilute *Nitricum acidum*. Mr. B. of a dark sallow complexion (note the unhealthy skin), aged 42, applied to me for a fistula-in-ano, which had existed for nearly a year, and which two of the best London surgeons agreed must be operated upon, saying it could not be cured without operation, he complained of soreness and burning pain in the lower bowel; a thin greenish discharge flowed freely from the fistula. I (Dr. Kidd) prescribed eight drops of dilute *Nitricum acidum* in a wine glass of water three times a day, without any local treatment. This perfectly and permanently cured the fistula in two months.'

This use of *Nitricum acidum* in fistula in ancient history with the homoeopaths. Hughes, 'Manual of Pharmacodynamics', third edition, well seems it up by pointing out that *Nitricum acidum* manifests great power over the mucocutaneous outlets, 'those parts where mucous membrane is exposed to the external air and where skin is so shielded and moistened that it approximates to mucous membrane' Hughes, writing still of *Nitricum acidum*, continues, 'It exhibits a singular power over the rectum and anus, it has cured prolaspus fistula and even fissure.'

Then Dr. Kidd gives (p. 175) the following:

Fistula-in-ano cured by *Hydrastis canadensis.*

'Mr L. aged 46, a Greek merchant came to me suffering from fistula-in ano, which had existed for three months. A well-known specialist and the family medical attendant assured him that he could not be cured without operation. Unwilling to submit to this he came to me. I prescribed ten drops of the tincture of *Hydrastis canadensis* in water, night and morning, also a compress over the fistula of four drachms of tincture of *Hydrastis canadensis* to four ounces of water applied on cotton wool, night and day'. To his great delight this perfectly cured him in a month. As our author gives no data or dates we cannot judge of the cases for ourselves, but they serve my purpose for quoting them, viz. to show that homoeopathy enables her followers to cure fistula medicinally and *Hydrastis canadensis* (as well as *Hydrastin*) is well known in the United States as possessing power over fistula-in-ano, and it is thence that we have both the remedy and our knowledge of it.

Hughes in his 'Manual of Therapeutics', writes of the medical cure of fistula as follows: 'Fistula-in-ano, you would hardly expect to be reached by internal remedies, and I am not confident that it would be so cured without local application also. But with the *Calendula officinalis* and *Hydrastis canadensis* of our Materia Medica thus applied we have several cases to report. There is one by Dr. Eadon in the 'Monthly Homeopathic Review' for June, 1865 in which *Calcarea phosphoricum*, with injections of *Calendula officinalis* lotion and the steam douche, proved curative; another by Mr. Clifton in the same journal for July, 1860, *Causticum* with *Calendula officinalis* being the remedies; and a third from America, in the 'British Journal' for October, 1868 where, *Nux vomica* and *Sulphur* were given with injections of *Hydrastin*. But, I am myself more than suspicious of the genuineness and the far reachingness of the cures by local applications. I do not mean that the cures reported are not genuine, but that the constitutional crisis underlying the fistular state can hardly be really cured by local remedies for

I do not believe that fistula is very often local in its nature, though it may be expressed in the anal region and nowhere else. The following from my own practice comes nearer my idea of a real cure:

## CASE OF FISTULA CURED BY MEDICINES

A stout middle-aged merchant came to me on April 20, 1887, for fistula-in-ano. His local medical man had got the fistula to heal by local and topical measures, but the uneasiness of the anal region was even greater than before. Patient had for long been subject to boils, but had had no complaints except measles and scarlatina in his childhood. From the fact that he had a good deal of pustular acne on certain parts of the body and also taking into account the fact that he had been twice vaccinated, I thought it likely that vaccinosis lay at the root of the disease expressed at the... anus.

The first remedy given was *Thuja occidentalis* 30, which was followed by a small lump at the part where the fistula had healed up, really it evidently was not. And there was another abscess just beginning. I then gave him *Bellis perennis* 1, five drops in water night and morning, and he thereafter had *Hepar sulphur* 3x, *Silicea terra* 6th trituration, and *Kalium cabonicum* 30, was then discharged perfectly cured. All the sclerosed circumanal tissue had become quite healthy, and his old eczema had also disappeared.

And I would remark that the disappearance of the eczema stamps the cure as like the disease, i. e., general and constitutional. And this is essentially important, for I much doubt whether the forcible healing up of fistula even by *Calendula officinalis* and *Hydrastis canadensis* or *Hydrastin*, or douches, is an unmixed advantage, unless the general state be simultaneously righted. For will anyone, on reflection, seriously tell me that fistula is even conceivable in a truly healthy individual? Big, stout men do indeed, get fistula, but are they truly healthy? I think not.

In 'L' Hahnemannisme' for October, 1872, Dr. Leon Simon reports as follows:

## FISTULA-IN-ANO

*Syphilinum* as injection, and charpie impregnated therewith, locally applied; internally, *Sulphur* 30, *Graphites* 30, *Silicea terra* 30 and 200, each remedy given successively for eight consecutive days, resulted in a cure in a few months. To this I would say: Why *Syphilinum*? It probably did no radical good, yet it serves to vitiate one's therapeutic conclusion. However, it is pleasing to note that our gallic colleagues cure fistula with medicines, and do not hack the poor sufferers about.

The more one's mind dwells upon the subject of fistula the less justifiable, nay, how utterly unsound does its surgical treatment appear. I used to have some valued friends among the surgeons, but I have long since offended them all with my outspokenness in regard to the comparatively humble handworker's sphere to which I would relegate what they are pleased to call the 'Science of Surgery'. I lost all my allopathic friends when I threw, in my lot with the peculiar therapeutic people called homoeopaths and have learned to do without them in my strong consciousness of right. Now I am beginning to learn to do without my chirurgical friends just because I can do without them, and so they cease to love me as of yore. Well, well, the pretty elastic ligature of my friends for *fistula-in-ano* is no more a cure for the fistular disease than is a catheter for the sclerosed state of the urethra, which we commonly call stricture.

*Berberis vulgaris*, a remedy very like *Hydrastis canadensis* has also cured fistula. Dr Schuessler, of Oldenburg, before he hatched his new duodecimal therapeusis, once wrote: 'Ich habe Mastdarmfistel mehrere Mal durch Berberis geheilt', but I suppose the tissue remedies have rendered *Berberis vulgaris* obsolete, if not inoperative, at least at Oldenburg.

I find a note on a fly-leaf of a book in my own handwriting, to the effect that Dr. Adams cured fistula with *Berberis vulgaris* 30.

Even old-school-surgeons are compelled to admit the amenability of fistula to medicinal and general treatment, though they make the admission rather shamefacedly, and as if yielding to vulgar prejudice. Thus the Messrs Allingham in 'Diagnosis and Treatment of Diseases of the Rectum' (a sound practical work from the merely mechanical standpoint), mention the subject of 'Cases cured by Treatment' with a contempt that I hardly think they can really feel. To speak of those who object to having their flesh cut about for fistula as 'wonderfully cowardly' is arrant nonsense. People with fistula are not well, else they would not have fistula, and my own idea is that having one's self cut for fistula is not a sign of courage, and still less of intelligence.

And I say this notwithstanding the dicta of all the great surgeons, special and general including my very distinguished friend Prof. Tod Helmuth, of New York. I tell them all that surgery is not needed as a rule for fistula, and even where it is unavoidable it is no cure. Of course, here and there a complete fistula with an opening which allows for the passage of feculent matter at frequent intervals; in such a case, naturally, the operation becomes unavoidable, but how often is that the case? Not at all often.

Allingham says (p.19):- 'When the fistula is complete, wind may pass through it and also faeces if the bowels are relaxed; as a rule, however, this symptom does not occur, in consequence of the smallness of the internal aperture, its situation, or its valvular form. It follows that, though the passage of wind is a certain indication of a complete fistula, the absence of this symptom should not induce the belief that there is no internal opening.'

Myself, I think, the reason why there is not usually any faecal discharge through a complete fistula, lies in the fact that the defecatory act twists and bends the fistular canal, and so occludes it more or less completely for the time being. Prof. Tod Helmuth ('System of Surgery', p. 779) thus treats of fistula from the standpoint of the physician.

## MEDICAL TREATMENT

When the inflammation is erysipelatous and spreads rapidly, *Belladonna* or *Rhus toxicodendron* may be prescribed. *Silicea terra* is a very important medicine, not only in the commencement of the affection, but also when the fistula is fully established. In the former case, if the abscess has not discharged, and the cellular membrane is found in a sloughty state, a free incision should be made to permit the escape or of the purulent secretion. If healthy action does not display itself, *Arsenicum album* and *China officinalis* must be prescribed.

*Mercurius solubilis, Sulphur, Silicea terra, Hepar sulphur* or *Calcarea carbonicum* must be exhibited if incarnation proceed imperfectly. If the constitution of the patient is impaired before operation is thought of appropriate medicines must be administered to eradicate any disease that may be present. In cases where the fistula has not been subjected to homeopathic treatment from the commencement, *Mercurius solubilis* or *Silicea terra* may be given. *Hepar sulphur* may be required after *Mercurius solubilis* when the fistula is extensive; and *Phosphorus* after *Silicea terra* where there is complication with disease of the lungs. When the digestive apparatus is impaired, *Calcarea carbonicum, Nux vomica, Mercurius solubilis,* and *Silicea terra* will prove valuable medicines.

*Causticum* is very important in cases of longstanding,

and in alternation with *Stlicea terra* I have known a fistula-in-ano to be healed for a time.

Dr. Eggert of Indianapolis and Dr. Grasmuck of Kansas, both report cases of fistula cured by internal medication, the latter gentleman using *Aesculus hippocastanum* cerate in connection with *Nux vomica* and *Sulphur*. My friend, Dr. Scriven, of Dublin, also related to me a successfully treated case.

Then Dr. Helmuth decides against the adequacy of remedies, and says surgical means must be resorted to as a general rule. On this point I very much question his power to speak with authority for the very reason that he is such a splendid surgeon. I well remember, some nine or ten years ago, Prof. Helmuth honouring me with a visit here, and showing me the then little known elastic ligature of Dittel, and so infectious was his enthusiasm for the thing that I really thought for a time medicines were nowhere. But some experience and mature reflection teach me that fistula cannot be really cured by any mechanical means whatsoever. Still, certain cases do need surgical aid, and then I cordially join Prof. Helmuth in his praise of the elastic ligature of Dittel. I say medicines first, and afterwards surgery if, unhappily, need be. There is a good practical work by Prof. J. S. Gilchrist ('Surgical Diseases and their Homeopathic Therapeutics', Chicago, 1880, third edition), from which I call the following practical cases, placed under the heads of the remedies used:

*Aloe socotrina*–A case is reported cured by Dr. Boyd ('Med. Invest.', vol. vi. p. 122), complicated with piles, in which the fistula was found cured when the piles had disappeared.

*Berberis vulgaris*–This remedy I have already referred to as curative of a certain kind of fistula. Dr. Admas (N. Y. State Socy. Trans., 1868, p. 378) gives a case cured with the following symptoms:-

Great soreness and pain throughout the entire back, from the sacrum to the shoulders, greatly increased from exercise. The fistula would close up, and inflammation and suppuration follow. Acrid leucorrhoeal discharge very prostrating.

*Lachesis mutus*–A case was cured in which, with other symptoms of the remedy, there was a full feeling of the rectum, and a sensation of little beating (Eggert, 'Med. Invest.', vol, vi. p, 143).

*Thuja occidentalis*- Eggert also reports a case cured with *Thuja occidentalis* in which the condylomatous condition was present.

*Arsenicum album*–Dr. Mera ('N. Y, Trans.', 1871.

p. 617) cured with *Arsenicum album* a case of fistula of ten years standing in which the symptoms were of great despondency, chills running up and down the back, relief from heat, large purple swelling in the right gluteal region.

*Causticum*–Gilchrist himself reports one case of fistula of one year's standing in an old man, very corpulent, the discharge being acrid, and accompanied with intense pruritus ani. The cure was speedy and radical.

Eggert's *Thuja occidentalis* case is rather better reported by Hoyle ('Clinical Therapeutics', vol. ii.) or rather Hoyle mentions two cases of fistula of the anus as having been cured by Eggert thus:

CASE–Two cases of blind external fistula with the symptoms at the verge of the anus & cauliflower excrescence of the size of a quarter of a dollar, and offensive perspiration around the parts affected. *Thuja occidentalis* 200, two doses, cured in ten weeks. Thus put, we understand the case better.

Eggert's *Lachesis mutus* case also requires a little more elucidation than Gilchrist Vouchsafes, viz., that the case was one of a lady at the climacteric. Put into the ordinary language of everyday clinical work, the *Thuja occidentalis* case was prescribed for on Hahnemann's recommendation as an anti-sycotic: the *Lachesis mutus*, because of the climacteric symptoms. Both successful cases and both treated according to the doctrines of Hahnemann in the Koethen phase of homeopathy.

The *Aloe socotrina* case was cured. The known effects of *Aloes socotrina* in haemorrhoids lead to its being prescribed. That is quite intelligible.

The indication in the *Berberis vulgaris* case was evidently the yellow leucorrhoeal discharge. In fact, primarily from the time old *signatura rerum naturalium* and the like may be said of *Thuja occidentalis* in sycosis.

Schuessler's use of *Berberis vulgaris* in fistula I have already mentioned.

In Ruckert's 'Klinische Erfahrungen' I find *Silicea terra** takes a very high rank.

1. A boy two years and a half old, was to be operated on for fistula, but two doses of Silicea cured it within three weeks – Altmuller.

2. A tender-skinned, fair-haired young man, in whom scabies had been twice got rid of with ointments,

_____

* Silicea was a favourite remedy with Hahnemann himself for fistula.

and who had been twice rid of gonorrhoea by injections, got an abscess in the perineum, near the anus, that had been opened surgically, but this would not heal up. The consequence was a fistula of the anus, accompanied with debility, emaciation, cough, and fever. Large doses of *China officinalis* were given to him in vain. His general condition was much ameliorated by *Sulphur*, and in about a week there was a tickling sensation at the aperture of the fistula, with an increased discharge of pure pus. *Sulphur* was repeated every sixth day. Afterwards three doses of *Silicea terra*, where upon the fistula was completely cured within three weeks from the time of its being first administered.

Here again we have the causal treatment in the first place, the prime antipsoric for psora.

Ruckert then mentions, at second hand, six cases of fistula-in-ano cured by Yeldham, and reported in the 'British Journal of Homeopathy.' but the remedies are not given.

In the 'Transactions of the Homoeopathic Medical Society of the State of New York', vol. ix., 1871, Dr. Alfred K. Hills makes (interalia) the following remarks, to which I partially subscribe:

*Hamamelis virginiana* in fistula—A certain physician, in prescribing for a patient, remarked that it was strange he could not hit the case, for rarely a patient came to him the third time without some relief. After racking his brain for a moment, he says, 'this case must be one of diseases of the intestinal canal, so I will give *Nitrate of silver.*' It is evident that the prescription was made upon a supposed pathological condition alone, and not upon the totality of the symptoms. In one of our journals is reported a case of fistula-in-ano. It is stated that the case was treated by a physician prejudiced ill favour of high potencies, who failed to ascertain the pathological condition, and there was no improvement under his statement. The writer says that when the case came into his hands, and examination revealed what he expected, viz. fistula, *Hamamelis virginiana* 1 was prescribed, and shortly the case was cured. Now, what do we gain by the statement that *Hamamelis virginiana* is good for fistula-in-ano? and shall we prescribe it for every such pathological condition? I cannot see that we add in the slightest degree to our knowledge of therapeutics by such generalization, and if we expect *Hamamelis virginiana* to cure every case of fistula-in-ano we shall be sadly disappointed. A patient presents himself to us suffering from headache, and states that it is made much worse from motion; now, when we hear this key-note, we must not feel satisfied that *Bryonia alba* is the remedy from this characteristic symptom, for whoever prescribes upon one subjective symptom will find himself as much mistaken, many times, as the man who prescribes upon one objective symptom, or the morbid anatomy and pathological show alone, regardless of the others, instead of the totality of the symptoms.

*Bryonia alba* will not cure every case of disease aggravated by motion, for other remedies have the same symptoms (*Belladonna, Nux vomica, Sanguinaria canadensis*), neither will *Hamamelis virginiana* cure every case of fistula-in-ano, for there are a number of remedies possessing marked symptoms in this direction.

What Dr. Hills here says is what I am trying to say throughout this little treatise, viz., that there is fistula and fistula, and what will cure one will not cure another.

The real reason, however, why for instance *Hamamelis virginiana* will not cure every case of fistula-in-ano is not because there are a number of remedies possessing marked symptoms in this direction, but because the fistular state or disease is not qualitatively (aetiologically and pathologically) the same in all persons having fistula. *Hamamelis virginiana* will cure the *Hamamelis virginiana* like fistular complaint, because like cures like, and when the fistular state of an individual is *Silicea terra* like, of course *Hamamelis virginiana* is no good, but *Silicea terra* is the remedy, and also conversely. But *Hamamelis virginiana* would also not cure all cases of fistula, even though we had no other remedy whatever possessing marked symptoms in this direction. Homoeopathicity to the case to be cured is the pharmacological desideratum here as elsewhere.

Moreover, there is another point to which I would direct attention. Dr. Hills says, 'The writer says that when the case came into his hands, an examination revealed what he expected, viz., fistula. *Hamamelis virginiana* 1 was prescribed, and shortly the case was cured. Now what do we gain by the statement that *Hamamelis virginiana* is good for fistula-in-ano and shall we prescribe it for every such pathological condition? I cannot see that we add in the slightest degree to our knowledge of therapeutics by such generalizations, and if we expect *Hamamelis virginiana* to cure every case of fistula-in-ano, we shall be sadly disappointed.'

Now, I think we gain a great deal when we know that, for instance *Hamamelis virginiana* can cure fistula-in-ano. In the first place, we gain the positive knowledge that, at least sometimes fistula-in-ano can be cured by medicines. We gain thus a direct proof of the truth of the general proposition as to the medicinal curability of fistula. Is that nothing? Let those who suffer from fistula decide, and further more, we gain the very important information that Hamamelis must stand in the list of our medicines of fistula. This must necessarily be always our first point de depart in all drug therapeutics. What Dr. Hills should say is this: 'We want to know not only that *Hamamelis virginiana* will cure fistula, but we also must know what constitutes the special indications for its use, so that we may know when to use it.' I enter into the point because this kind of seemingly sapient, yet really shallow criticism is often levelled against published cases of cure. We must of course, aim at the bull's eye of fine pharmic differentiations, but if we do not begin to shoot till we can certainly hit the bull's eye, we shall never hit the therapeutic bull's eye at all.

Your superfine critic is commonly very sterile himself. I fancy I once read in a copy book, *Pour BIEN parler, il faut commencer par MAL parler.*

*Solanum nigrum* is recommended as a local application in most fistulas. This quality of it no doubt has in common with so many of the other solanaceous plants.

*Aurum metallicum* in Fistulas–Just ten years ago I published a small volume on the general use of this great remedy, entitled 'Gold as a remedy in Disease, etc.' (pp. 106, 107). Pliny already speaks of it (qy. in ana?).

Case of fistula-in-ano–Young man, twenty-one years of age, bilious-sanguine temperament. For five months fistula-in-ano, excrescences on scrotum (eight months after primary symptoms). Cured with five grains of the perchloride of *Gold*; all the symptoms had disappeared with the third grain (Clinique of M. Lallemand, in Legrand. p. 188)

Another young man of bilious temperament, twenty-six years old, of strong constitution had chancres, fistula-in-ano, for five months.

He was cured with five grains of the perchloride of *Gold*. In that kind of anal fistula for which *Kalium carbonicum* is such a classic remedy, *Aurum metallicum* does not suggest itself to my mind, but rather in that dependent upon a specific taint, and notably after *Mercurius solubilis*.

Prof. E. M. Hale ('Homeopathic Materia Medica

of the New Remedies', 1867) mentions *Collinsonia canadensis, Hydrastis canadensis* and *Sanguinaria canadensis* as probable remedies in fistula of the anus.

Of *Phytolacca decandra* Hale says: 'Dr. Paine (eclectic), after asserting that the *Phytolacca decandra* will cause burning in stomach, tenderness of the bowels, heat in the rectum, tenesmus, and bloody discharges, dysentery and haemorrhoids gives his experience in its use. I have treated a large number of cases of ulceration of the rectum with remarkable success. A physician of note who had treated himself, and had been treated by others with all the ordinary remedies for what was called a cancerous affection of the rectum, applied to me some two years since, and I placed him upon one-half grain doses of *Phytolaccinum* every two or three hours, together with nutritious diet and an enema of warm water every day. This treatment was continued for two or three months, and resulted in a complete cure.'

Fissure, prolapsus recti, and piles have also been cured by *Phytolacca decandra.* Prof. Hale compares it to *Nitricum acidum* and *Mercurius solubilis* and probably few men know more of drug action than does Hale.

## CASE OF FISTULA-IN-ANO

On May 17, 1889, an unmarried city gentleman thirty years of age, came under my observation for fistula-in-ano. Four or five years previously he had an abscess on the edge of the anus. It burst and healed. Fourteen months ago another one in the same spot. It burst with the aid of poulticings, and healed up. Some moisture and blood ooze therefore ever since. Patient is dusky and delicate looking. On examination, I found a small opening to an incomplete fistula. He also complained of feverishness and indigestion.

R

*Tc. Pyrogenium* 5, five drops in water night and morning.

May 31-'I am much better.' How do you know?

'Because the sweating at my seat that I had for so many years has gone.' Complains that in warm weather he is apt to get dry eczema of the hands. Since taking the *Pyrogenium* his skin has assumed a cleaner aspect.

*Thuja occidentalis* 30 in infrequent dose.

June 29-Discharged thick matter and blood soon after beginning with the powders. The fistula still discharges, and there is a good deal of sclerosed tissue at its bottom and around it. Patient is dusky and drowsy.

℞

*Nux vomica* 1x, five drops in water night and morning.

August 7-Perfectly well of the fistula, and of the circumjacent telar sclerosis. Just before the fistula began to heal up definitely, a small calculus, hard and sharp, size of a pea was passed from it with much pain, or rather it pained very much, and on feeling the part he discovered the calculous formation and removed it, and brought it to me.

## CASE OF POITRINARY FISTULA

This designation of fistula in connection with chest symptoms seems to me convenient, and I accordingly coin it.

A city gentleman, single, thirty-five years of age, came to me on March 4, 1889, for fistula-in-ano and chest. He informed me that he had had much expectoration of phlegm all his life, but for the past two years the same had become bloody. For a number of years, under homoeopathic treatment with benefit, he had maintained his ground, and even gained a little in strength and bulk. Present weight ten stone. I found his throat studded with tubercles, his lungs very flat, vocal

resonance much increased at both apices, and all down
the left side of the thorax; he is very shortwinded,
coughs and expectorates almost incessantly; his skin is
dingy, dusky and greasy; the glands of his neck hard,
though small; the phlegm is thick, yellow-green. For
the past two years has been suffering from fistula.
Under my treatment the old fistula dried up, but then
(Ap. 9) a new one formed on the other side. Previously,
he had been twice cut for fistula. This needless torture
I was able to spare him.

April 29-Perineal abscess reopened, burst,
discharged very freely, and has now all healed.

May 13-Fistula quite well.

August 9-Fistula continues well. Patient himself
much better and stronger, and remains under treatment
for his throat and chest. Patient received some nosodes–
*Thuja occidentalis* 30, *Hydrastis canadensis* θ, *Nux
vomica* lx, and *Dulcamara* θ.

I have myself not met with many cases of fistula in
the very young, but here is one.

## FISTULA IN AN INFANT

On June 23, 1879, a country gentleman brought his
little six-year old son to me for fistula-in-ano. At its

birth the nurse discovered a lump at the seat. A little time afterwards this gathered and burst like a boil, and had continued ever since to gather and burst at intervals. The right eye had no lashes; he had severe ophthalmia tarsi of the same eye also ever since he was born.

An examination of the anal region showed a fistula external and incomplete and numerous scars where others had healed. The right nostril was also chronically inflamed. If he gets a thorn or splinter in his flesh, it festers as does equally the tiniest scratch or prick. A connection between eye and fistula is noticed. For when the eye is very bad the anus gets better and conversely.

R

*Tc. Phosphorus* 30 three drops in water night and morning.

July 24-The eye-lashes are beginning to grow.

R

*Tc. Kalium carbonicum* 30.

October 20-Fistula cured. His nose bothers him a good deal, becoming very much inflamed. There is considerable matter discharge from the eye.

R

*Aurum foliatum* 3 trituration, four grains dry on the tongue twice a day.

January 15, 1880-Fistula continues well; nose well; eye better, lashes perceptibly growing.

Repeat the *Aurum foliatum*, but in the fourth centesimal trituration, four grains at bed-time only.

July 25, 1881-Fistula and nose continue well; there is now quite a show of eye-lashes; still some ophthalmia tarsi, however around the meatus of the left ear there is some eczema.

R

*Psorinum* 30 in infrequent dose, and thereafter *Thuja Occidentalis* 30 in like manner.

Discharged quite cured.

Four years later he was again brought, but this time for enlarged tonsils, which our ordinary remedies slowly (not rapidly) cured, and then he was reported well, and I again ascertained that he was well in all respects in February 1894.

It is not often that one meets with fistula in the very young. The eye, nose, and anal troubles all yielded to remedies administered internally and the permanency thereof proved by nearly fifteen years of subsequent observation.

I suppose the 'proper' treatment of this case would have been–

Firstly, an operation for the fistula by a specialist for the anal affection.

Secondly, the eye must have been treated by an oculist, who would have used his greases and his washes, and the never-lacking *Nitras argenti*.

Thirdly, the eczema must have been treated by a skin-doctor also, without any doubt, with an ointment.

Fourthly, the nose must have specially needed the services of a rhinologist.

Fifthly, the enlarged tonsils would have afforded an opportunity for the exercise of the special skill of a throat specialist, who would have whipped off the tonsils by an operation never before invented.

And, finally, as the good lad was nervous, and twitched once or twice a moon, do doubt his prepuce would have been ablated or slit open. Quite lately a noble peer told me gleefully that he had just had his son circumcised, and also had had his tonsils removed, and I fear his Lordship thought me rude when I replied that the Creator must have bungled a good deal, else why these needless tonsils and superfluous prepuces?

It is satisfactory to note that some of the greater physician are beginning to see the true effects of specialism.

Thus, I lately read an account of the Eighth Medical Congress at Wiesbaden, and in it the following report summarized from the 'Berliner klin. Wochenschrift' Nos. 18 and 19, 1889:

Herr Petersen (Copenhagen) read an important paper 'On the Hippocratic Method of Treatment', or, in other word, 'On Hippocratism'. Although this mode of treatment seemed overdrawn in many respects, many of its principles were still deserving of recognition. Hippocrates' designation of fever as *instrumentum felicissimum* was now seen to be worthy of praise. With Hippocrates the whole man was ill, not one particular organ only; hence specialism was excluded. An extremely individual treatment was adopted. The first aim of treatment was not scientific, but sanative, and the chief means were dietetic. The physician was a 'healing artist' who became such only by unwearied diligence and powerful talent, especially the gift of observation. The whole cultivation was mainly clinical. The French had become more anatomical, while the English remained true to 'Hippocratism'. In Germany, medicine, as directed by Trauble, Rokitansky, and Virchow, had departed from Hippocratism; but since then, under the influence of Fredrichs and Leyden, seemed inclined to return to it. Modern medicine must return to the ancient path, or it would be destroyed by specialism.

## PILES, PERINEAL ABSCESSES AND FISTULA

One certainly meets with a goodly number of cases of fistula in portly men about forty years of age. Such is one, a dark gentleman, forty-one years of age, came under my observation on November 26, 1887, complaining of his liver and perineal abscess, and also haemorrhides. Patient suffered also from pains in the stomach, coming on in the early morning about six or seven o'clock. Both liver and spleen were swelled, tongue and fingers gouty, slight eczema of anal region and there was much depression of spirits, attributed to business worries.

R

*Nux vomica* lx, five drops in water, night and morning.

February 4, 1888 - Much better in almost all respects; only had the stomach pains once lately. Complains of anal irritation on getting warm in bed at night. Sleeps badly; has much business worry, and is in consequence depressed; weight on the top of the head.

R

*Sulphur* 30.

May 5-Not very materially improved: has indigestion, anal irritation, insomnia, depression of spirits, some uncomfortable feelings about the heart, and he has grown very stout of late.

R

*Tc. Vanadium ammonium* 12.

Feb. 16, 1889-Has had another perineal abscess, and there is now an incomplete external fistula with much mattery discharge.

Two months of *Phytolaccinum* 3x, six grains at bed-time, cured him of the fistula, and he was otherwise so far well that he did not want my further treatment.

## SYMPATHETIC RELATIONS BETWEEN THE ANUS AND THE HEAD

One very frequently observes an intimate sympathy between the anal region and the head. Let me relate a case in point. A gentleman of sixty was under my care for haemorrhoids and nocturnal pruritus ani that at times was maddening, and which had worried him for many years, and for the cure of which an almost endless array of local applications had been used in vain. He used to have attacks of giddiness and faintings, and he also had a small lipoma in the poll. What distressed him most was the *pruritus ani*, due, he thought, to threadworms. My treatment cured his giddiness, but the anal itchings grew rather worse than better. I will here interpolate the remark that whisky often causes itchings at the seat at night, and then the cure consists in leaving off the whisky. But this gentleman did not take whisky, being a teetotaller for many years.

The only time in his life he had ever obtained a respite from his pruritus was from the cure at Kissingen, so to Kissingen he would go, though I tried to dissuade him from it.

The Kissingen cure was effectual, for he returned without the pruritus ani. However not every long after his return from Kissingen, cured of the pruritus, he had a fit, consisting in a long fainting attack, evidently cephalic, and he became very giddy and habitually unsteady in his gait, so that he was afraid to go about. Moreover he then got partial ptosis, notably of the left side. In this state he returned under my care. *Zincum aceticum* put his head quite right, and he feels now perfectly well and sure of gait, and free from faintings, and the ptosis is better, but the nightly itchings at the anus have returned. For these and for the lump in the neck which, however, is decreased he remains under my treatment, I should say that patient carries on an enormous business, and often sits up half the night intensely occupied with intricate calculations, while on sunday he takes a complete rest in the form of preaching and Sunday-school teaching. He is a grand man, but whether the Master's work, at this time of day, needs such a sacrifice may be questioned. My own opinion is that a labourer is worthy of his rest.

But my point here is the sympathy between the anal region and the head.

By the way, for a fagged brain *Zincum aceticum* lx, five drops in water night and morning, is indeed mighty for good (See: Rademacher's experiment in 'Erfahrungsheillehre')

## PROLAPSUS AND THREATENED FISTULA

A gentleman consulted me last summer in a very agitated frame of mind for fistula. An examination of the parts disclosed slight rectal prolapse, and a certain amount of inflammation of the projecting folds of the mucous membrane lining the rectum, in which the haemorrhoidal vessels were very prominent. He had

been operated on for fistula, and also for piles and
prolapse; but notwithstanding all this beautiful rectal
surgery, the unfortunate patient is never comfortable at
the seat nor do I think he ever will be, as the anal region
is puckered with the crookedly healed tissue, and a
blind funnel has been produced more than half an inch
deep; this funnel is lined with common integument,
and would otherwise be an incomplete fistula. There
was blood at the anus almost every day. His nerves
had received a grave shock from the operations, for
notwithstanding the ten years that had elapsed since
they were performed he still suffers from the effects. I
have often been struck with the grave head symptoms
that occur at the same time as rectal troubles, and
these former are made much worse by all surgical
interference. Thus this gentleman lives in a constant
state of daze and fright lest a further operation should
be needful for piles, prolapse, or fistula; his so called
nervous headaches are at times so bad that he thinks he
will go out of his mind. The very mention of the words
'fistula' or 'prolapse' quite horrifies him.

A close examination showed so little to account
for his state, that I was led to conclude that his very
numerous vaccinations might have caused his trouble,
he had been vaccinated five times.

Remedies greatly improved his condition, and so far that there was no further fear of fistula. *Thuja occidentalis* was the principal remedy; infrequent doses of the thirtieth dilution administered during two months. He is not comfortable at the seat, nor do I think he ever will be, a fact due, I think, to the bungling way in which he had been operated on. I see evidences of bungling after operations in this region so very seldom that I am constrained to admit this much in common fairness to the surgeons, that they believe in the operations I do not doubt; that they do their work well I can testify; but that their views are erroneous and their practice bad I am certain.

## TUBERCULOUS FISTULA BY INFECTION

A certain number of cases of anal fistula in middle-aged, highly-nourished men come under my observation, and I have been struck with the fact that their wives had either died of, or were suffering from, consumption. Four such cases in one year have I observed, and I have been constrained to ask myself the question, whether these cases do not represent a class by themselves? The frequent coincidence deserves at least some attention. I would not be too hasty in generalizing, but anyone who sees much of fistula may, I think, readily verify the fact for themselves. I imagine that the fistula represents, in such cases, an infection from a consumptive wife communicated to the husband in the intimate relations of married life. I commend the subject to the consideration of my colleagues. I imagine, further, that the infected husbands, had they been prone to phthisis of the tuberculous variety, would in all probability have developed genuine consumption, but not being so prone, they simply maintain a tuberculous sore-the fistula-in-ano much as one observes obstinate tuberculous sores on parts exposed to mechanical infection from cuts and the like, as, for instance, on the hands, whereof numerous cases are on record in general medical literature. I take it that the infection is truly tuberculous in the bacillary sense, but the soil is not fit; the constitutional power is too great to allow of the development of general tuberculosis.

That this kind of locally limited tuberculous infection does actually exist, I am satisfied. One sees this also exemplified at rare intervals in syphilis. In certain very obstinate cases of Hunterian chancres that becomes very unusually penetrating with a distinct resistance to specific treatment that is otherwise usually successful, and that promptly, I have of late been led to assume the existence of a tuberculous mother soil, and have treated the two pathological states simultaneously, and at any rate they begin forthwith to mend. I will relate a very instructive case in point.

## URINARY FISTULA-A REMARKABLE CASE

Some seven years since, a London professional man came under my observation for an ordinary gonorrhoea. He is otherwise a good, conscientious fellow, but harvested the wages of sin at the very start, and was in a great state of mental perturbation. I was, after careful examination, enabled to assure him that he had a gonorrhoeal urethritis, and nothing else; there was absolutely no sign or suspicion of anything beyond that. *Aconitum napellus*, *Hepar sulphur*, *Hydrastis canadensis* and *Cynosbati* were administered, and in some six or seven weeks I thought were out of the wood, there only a little urethral suintement left. But one day, without any concern whatever, he told me he thought, he had caught a cold, and was getting a boil in the fork, that he also had some lumps in the groin, and nettle rash on the body. The experienced may judge of my utter amazement when I discovered a typical roseola syphilitica all over his body, notably on the chest and abdomen, and all the superficial glands of the body enlarged and indurated. Moreover, on the under surface of the member, some two inches or more from its extremity, and just in front of the prostate there was in the very deed a 'boil' of the size of a gooseberry, and very hard. I set to work vigorously with antisyphilitic treatment, and in a few weeks the roseola and other prominent symptoms had much abated, but his hair came out, and the nuchal glands were very prominently enlarged. During all this time the urethral discharge, which had returned, persisted. Just as I thought I was mastering both the gonorrhoea and the syphilis, he called one day and informed me that he had a leak in the region of the boil (as said boil had burst). *Horrible dietu.* I found a fully established urethral fistula, with a thick hard wall surrounding and lining it. Several further months of persistent treatment finally resulted in a cure of the gonorrhrea and of most of the manifestations of syphilis, but the terrible fistula persisted, notwithstanding *Mercurius solubilis, Aurum metallicum, Nitricum acidum, Stillingia silvatica, Iodium,* and *Silicea terra* and some other seemingly likely remedies. I do not easily despair of a case, but when distinct consumptive symptoms began to show themselves, I certainly felt very anxious indeed and I deemed it my duty to tell my poor patient that I feared he would have to undergo an operation for the urinary fistula, as it, seemed to be wearing him out. However. I thought the matter over a few days, and finally came to the conclusion that the fistula was not only syphilitic, but also tuberculous, though how the infection could have been communicated within the urethra some three inches from the orifice I cannot even now understand. I then alternated *Mercurius solubilis Hahnemanni* 3x with very infrequent doses of *Bacillinun* C. (six grains of the former, and as many globules of the latter to the dose). At the same time I put him on very full diet with a generous wine.

*Result*-In a few months the patient was quite well in every respect. The indurated glands all returned to the normal, the hair grew again, the night-sweats ceased, the fistula completely healed up, the sclerosis around it disappeared, and patient put on flesh and reassumed his old healthy appearance.

I will finish this long story by remarking that the amelioration, that set in as soon as he was put on the last mentioned double prescription, was truly remarkable, and for weeks and weeks whenever it was discontinued for other remedies, the amelioration at once ceased, so that I had to refer to it over and over again. The *Bacillinum* was, however, never given more than one dose in four days. The *Mercurius solubilis* three times a day. To look at this gentleman now no one would suspect what he has gone through. *Aux grands maux les grands remedes*, they say over in France. This case forcibly reminds one of Hunter's famous experiment on himself. We have here a case of urinary fistula, a very bad one too, and its having been perfectly and permanently cured with medicines, should encourage us all to treat urinary fistulas also with medicines only, a thing I believe never even attempted. Perhaps I had better add, to prevent mistakes or misapprehension, that absolutely no local applications were used, not even a bit of lint or charpie.

I do not think it would serve any useful end where I were to detail any more cases of fistula, as I think I have proved my point: *fistula can be cured medicinally*.

## GENERAL REFLECTIONS ON FISTULA

Fistula is practically just a convenient term for a certain morbid state found at a given part, and it cannot be regarded as a disease sui generis though it is itself a generic term which potentially includes quite a number of diseases of a more or less formidable nature.

Fistula is a condition that is sequential to another condition, viz., to a gathering or abscess of some kind, and when we speak of a fistula say a fistula-in-ano we mean that at the indicated part there is a variously shaped, often a pipe-shaped, mattering portion of eroded or otherwise denuded tissue. Now it is commonly taught that this discharging pipe-like abscess is in itself the disease, and that its cure consists in cutting it open, cleaning it, and making it heal, and there the thing is supposed to end.

But is it so?

I know a lady who in 1868 was abroad, and suffering from fistula, and the local family doctor ordered her home to London to be operated on for her fistula, he having previously tried divers local applications in vain. She came home to London and was operated on, and cured-that is to say, the fistula with a good deal of trouble was got to heal up. After that the *os uteri* became gravely ulcerated and patient spent nearly two years for the most part lying on her back, and underwent an almost endless number of local manipulations and operations. At length the ulcerations in the region of the os were made to heal. Then came leucorrhoea without ulceration and of a most distressing kind; a very dapper gynaecologist occupied several years in stemming this discharging tide, and when the unfortunate lady had been fairly rid of the leucorrhoea by the injections so long and so strong, she found herself cured surgically and completely of firstly of fistula-in-ano; secondly of ulceration of the os uteri; and thirdly, and lastly of this severe leucorrhoea. And then? health? Not at all, but a hard tumour in the region of bowel and womb, which has rendered her state simply awful; for, apart from the ultimate significance of the tumour *per se*, the exit of the bowel being almost obliterated, that going to stool can be only characterized as awful, so distressing, so tedious and so painful.

Now, what is the meaning of this all? Just this, the lady was ill in herself, and her organism tried to rid itself of some of (at least) the product of her ill-being, to this end it constructed a fistula in an out of the way district of the economy, through which it might drain off matter inimical to itself. The surgeons, in forcibly healing the fistula practically stopped the outlet pipe. Then the same process was repeated in regard to the said ulceration and again with the surface outlet, which we call leucorrhoea and finally finding all direct outlets effectually blocked by the doctors. Nature was fairly compelled to deposit within the organism the before mentioned inimical matter in the form of a tumour and that at the next nearest available point to the seat of the fistula, ulcers and leucorrhoea respectively. Controvert this, ye men – of the knife, if ye can.

## FISTULA AND LEUCORRHOEA

We have just seen that when the fistula was closed forcibly, leucorrhoea took its place. Now one comes across notable examples of cases supposedly of leucorrhoea which turn out to be chronic fistula, the diapers and linen being taken as evidence of the said leucorrhoea. I myself treated a case of very severe fistula for a considerable time mistaking it for leucorrhoea, no examination having been made. It is not always easy to tell when and whether it is our duty to make a proper examination of the anal and crural regions in ladies. Fortunately it is quite possible to treat the one, and yet cure the other. This may sound very odd to the uninitiated, but it is really a high compliment to the method of treatment in as much as it shows that, in all probability, the patient was being treated, and not the name merely of her disease, for she was also cured. I went by the symptoms and state of the patient, and principally by the tongue, by the tint of the skin, and by the nature of the discharge, and though I was needlessly long about it, still the lady made a perfect recovery, and remains well to this day. The amount of the discharge was at one time very great. The principal remedies used were *Thuja occidentalis*, *Hydrastis canadensis*, *Sepia officinalis*, *Chelidonium majus*, *Hepar sulphur*, *Silicea terra*, *Psorinum*, *Sabina* and *Aqua silicata*. A brother of this lady is being wrecked by fistula for notwithstanding several operations and the very best hygiene, the surgeons say the fistula will not heal; the poor conceited ignoramus himself thinks homoeopathy 'very well for women and children' (in which he is right), but no use in fistula.

Here, I would like to ask the fistula cutters how it is that (the fistula being as they contend, of local origin and nature), when they fail to force the healing-up process, they then say that the fistula will not heal. Leucorrhoea is a constitutional disorder; so is fistula; and they are not infrequently of absolutely identical nature and significance, though, of course, they just as often differ so much that they have nothing in common but their ill fate of constituting the happy hunting ground of specialists 'of the world worldly, of the earth earthy.'

## THE PRE-FISTULAR ABSCESS

When a certain limited portion of tissue stagnates in its circulatory life, it dies, and must be got rid of. Nature cuts off its blood supply and it dies and when the circumscribed mortification of the tissue is sufficiently advanced, the abscess bursts and discharges, and if there be no morbid *vis a tergo*, the abscess begins to heal and Nature is not very long in mending the lesion in the continuity of her tissues.

One sees the whole philosophy of the thing. Nature's simple and yet, adequate way of working. When a foreign body is in the living tissue and Nature sets about turning the intruder out. I have often watched the process, as no doubt most people have. It is simply this: take the case of a thorn driven into the tissue of the hand and breaking off; there is first the lesion, then the foreign body–the broken off thorn. Next we have heat, pain, redness, and swelling the classic calor, dolor, rubor, tumor; then the outermost portion dies, becomes purulent, rotten, the foreign body is then expelled slowly at the mattering dead spot or point. If there be an obstacle to its exit the whole, just described process keeps on repeating itself, there is a burrowing process which is continued until a point of exit is reached or failing the possibility of this, Nature will at times encapsule it. But, assuming the possibility of an easy exit, the process is not a long one, and as soon as the foreign body is got rid of, Nature needs no further help (the individual being normally or even only fairly healthy), but forth with mends the gap in the tissues by carnification, and there is an end of it, only the young newly carnified tissue being very vascular will remain for a time red, until, in fact, the new vascular loops (being no longer needed) atrophy. Thus the foreign body being ejected, and the gap made by its passage mended by carnification (healed up), there is nothing more to be said, the affair is at an end.

But it is not thus with the pre-fistular abscess, and therefore necessarily not thus with the fistula itself: here we have to do, not only with the morbid matter (stuff) that caused the abscess, but with an internal abscess and fistula causing disease that is more or less constantly at work, and the product of this disease requires an outlet which the prefistular abscess was meant to prepare, and which is represented by the fistula. Had Nature got rid of all the morbid product the exit would no longer be needed, and the fistula would very soon heal up of itself, as the saying goes. Everybody knows that if he gets a thorn into his flesh, and he forthwith pulls it out entire and entirely, he is spared the relatively long and round about process that Nature adopts if it is left in, and which we have just attempted to describe, a good surgeon, therefore, in all cases seeks to get at the intruded foreign body and extract it. But the surgeon seeks in other processes to come to Nature's aid, and instead of waiting for an abscess to mature and burst, he makes a free incision and lets out the pus or what not. Now, where there is an obstacle to its exit (such as a fascia) this is no doubt not only good practice, but is imperative to prevent needless tissue destruction, burrowing, and the formation of sinuses, with the concomitant fever, pain, and exhaustion. But where there is no great obstacle in the way of a spontaneous bursting. I feel very sure that it is best not to incise, but to let the boil ripen and burst, and in the meantime 'go for' the cause of the said boil by treating the patient with the proper remedies. When this is successfully done, and the boil bursts of itself, the discharge is more free, and the consequent organismic depuration more complete.

On this effort of Nature to rid herself of noxious substances a system of treatment by manipulation has been furnished, and which has been named *Kellgrenism* in honour of its discoverer Kellgren. This system has an organ of its own called *The Tocsin*, edited by Dr. Frederick A. Fleyer, a man of very great ability and learning. From its issue of September 1, 1889, I take their own account of the system, because it fits into my subject at this point.

## TREATMENT BY MANIPULATION*

In a previous issue we have endeavoured to give some idea of the nature and object of medical exercises and we are now anxious to show the nature and object of treatment by manipulation for the cure of disease.

In the first place, it must be remembered that all alteration in the normal condition of the body, that is to say, all forms of disease, cause the formation of morbid substances of some kind or another. The nature of these morbid products together with the conditions which give rise to them, are too technically scientific to be dealt with in this article suffice it to say, that these products are, roughly speaking, either what is commonly known as matter and gas. The formation of these naturally cause obstruction in the parts affected, to the detriment more or less of the whole system. It is equally obvious, therefore, that these obstructions must be got rid of before health can be restored.

---

*This article may be taken as illustrating the Kellgren philosophy and treatment of disease.

Where matter has formed, as in the case of wounds, abscesses, etc., it may be removed by working it to the surface and giving it an outlet there, and by dispersion. Most people can see the value of gently pushing matter towards the wound or boil, but many are apt to regard dispersion with disfavour. If matter has formed they say, it is far better to encourage it to tend towards the one centre, where it can discharge, than to spread the evil all over the body by backening it. *It must be remembered, however, that matter is not a foreign body which has been somehow introduced into the system; on the contrary, it is a collection of legitimate products (in the first instance) which have become disorganized. As dirt has been defined as 'matter out of place', so the morbid products of the body are legitimate constituents of the organism unlawfully congregated together. The white corpuscles of the blood, for instance, form bad matter, although they are healthy and necessary constituents of the blood when they move in a legitimate manner. To disperse these, and to force them back to their proper spheres is not to spread matter over the body, therefore, but to dissolve it into its original elements.* Where morbid products have been formed for some time however, processes of putrefaction ensue which render it impossible to disperse it, because the elements themselves become diseased, and it is then necessary to cause their discharge from the body. The task of deciding which method of treatment to apply is not so difficult as may be supposed, since Nature to a great extent decides the question herself. Where a wound or abscess is already formed, and shows itself plainly, it is probable that putrefaction has taken place and, therefore, the great aim should be to promote its discharge, but if this stage has not been reached, it is sufficient simply to manipulate the place affected thus causing movement in the obstructed tissues. If the elements of which the matter is composed are still healthy, the manipulation will loosen them from their position and drive them to their proper places; but if putrefaction has already begun, it will drive it to the surface, where it has the best chance of getting free. It must be borne in mind that Nature is always trying to rid herself of unhealthy products, and manipulation, by encouraging movement in congested parts, assists the blood to throw off the poison which infects it, and drives it for refuge to the surface, which it will then try to burst through.

In most diseases it is gas and not matter which forms the obstruction. This gas, which, like matter, is also a natural product of the body increases too much in volume, and is altered in its nature by any deviation from the normal state of health, and forms a swelling, often imperceptible, in that part of the body where the disease has originated. This swelling can easily be detected by trained fingers and is very sensitive to the touch. This power of detecting where a disease lies with the fingers is of the utmost value, because pain is often reflex and gives no clue to the real seat of the malady. It also stands to sense that if a cure by manipulation is to be effected, the manipulator must be allowed to use his or her own discretion as to the places which are to be worked upon. It is nonsense for a patient to say, work on my head for headache, or on my limb for rheumatism; there is no occasion to touch any other part of my body as I am quite well otherwise. A person's digestion may seem sound for instance, because the form of indigestion from which they suffer shows itself indirectly by some reflex pain in the head or the limbs. To work at these only may give temporary relief, but no cure can reasonably be expected from such a partial method of treatment.

The actual nature of manual treatment is either that of making frictions with the fingers or by vibrations. In no case are the fingers moved about over the skin, as in rubbing; the frictions and vibrations are made through the skin on nerves and vessels etc., It is moreover, quite unnecessary to work upon the bare skin, a certain amount of loose clothing being no obstacle whatever to the efficacy of the work.

I give the article entire, so that I may be quite fair. That the Kellgren treatment by manipulation is a close imitation of Nature is clear and it must therefore command our respectful consideration, particularly when defended by such an able advocate as Dr. Floyer, whose writings in *The Tocsin* are a delight to read. But I have thus far seen no published results and have consequently nothing to judge it by as a practical system of curative medicine. Awaiting these I suspend judgment.

What is matter?

By the word matter is here meant, not matter in a general scientific sense, but, say the contents of an abscess.

In the foregoing article I have italicised the following: '*It must be remembered, however, that matter is not a foreign body which has been somehow introduced into the system; on the contrary, it is a collection of legitimate products (in the first instance) which have become disorganized. As dirt has been defined as "matter out of place", so the morbid products of the body are legitimate constituents of the organism unlawfully congregated together. The white corpuscles of the blood, for instance, form bad matter, although they are healthy and necessary constituents of the blood when they move in a legitimate manner. To disperse these, and to force them back to their proper spheres is not to spread matter over the body, therefore, but to dissolve it into its original elements.'*

Now, let us examine these statements.

We may grant that matter is made up of the white blood corpuscles which have wandered out of the circulation, but why have they wandered out? Why did they not stay at home and live happily together in the blood? The reason is that they have become charged with a function, their mission has become a new one, and they wander out of the blood that is within the vessels in order to carry away a given poison, or virus, or other hurtful things, they are poisoned, and hurry out of the circulation *en masse* and hasten to a common rendezvous at the surface, to be cast out as matter. These blood corpuscles are no longer mere blood corpuscles, but poisoned members of their community, and they hasten out of the body to save it, they offer themselves a sacrifice on the altar of the organism. They are not runaway sinners run wild, as it were, in a herd. Not at all; on the contrary, they are so law-abiding that they sacrifice themselves to duty, and they are in numbers proportionate to the quantity of poison that has to be got rid of; the more the poison the greater the number of corpuscles. It follows, therefore, that to force these poison-carrying, out-wandered blood corpuscles back whence they came (if it were possible) must be bad practice indeed; and to do so would be backening the matter and spreading the poison of which they are the dying or dead carriers, all over the body.

Dr. Floyer says – 'The morbid products of the body are legitimate constituents of the organism unlawfully congregated together'. This is impossible; what he should say were a morbid product of the body is no longer a constituent of the organism at all. On the contrary, the erstwhile blood corpuscles having become morbid are cast out or wander out, and so cease to be constituents. The act of congregating together is merely their collective mode of exit from the economy.

The putrefactive process is a secondary affair. If the morbid products are dispersed, and sent back before the process of putrefaction sets in, then they carry back merely the poison they had brought out; while if they are sent back subsequent to putrefaction, then they may carry back with them not only the poison they were carrying away, but also products of the putrefaction.

I am, therefore, with those who regard dispersion with disfavour, particularly if the boil constituents are poison carriers, as I believe they usually are, and that notwithstanding the fact that the *boil-constituents* were previously *body-constituents*.

Finally, it seems to me that Kellgrenism is in itself contradictory, for while it is contended for it that it aids Nature to expel the peccant matter or gas, it is also maintained that it aids Nature by dispersing what Nature has gathered together. Both can only be tenable if it be held that the disorder consequent upon the obstructions to the circulation are synonymous with the disorders themselves.

It seems to me that if it be good to help Nature to bring the matter to the periphery and let it out, it cannot be good to disperse what Nature unaided had already brought together in a boil for ejectment. That is in general principle. Of course, if it can be shown that the disorder is primarily stagnation, and nothing else–say capillary stasis–then dispersion (early enough) and cure would be identical terms.

## THE LOCALIST'S POSITION CONTRADICTORY

The localistic surgeons, who claim that operation is a cure of fistula, tell us that the pre-fistular abscess must be opened to let the matter out, while the fistula must be operated upon to make it close. So, according to this, the essence of the disease in the case of the abscess lies in the fact that Nature cannot, unaided, get rid of the matter; while in the fistula, where she does get freely rid of the matter, the essence of the disease lies in the fact that Nature is helping herself.

The Kellgrenists seem to consider that stasis is the real factor in boils; for me, the stasis is merely a concomitant–just the first necessary stage in effecting an organic lesion of the peripheral continuity to gain an outlet for inimical stuff, be this stuff leucomaine, ptomaine, cadaverine, urea or even bacilli or microbes.

Abscess is not a disease *sui generis*; it is a patho-biological process, and we have, in each case of abscess, to consider this patho-biological process by itself, i.e., Nature's method of turning out an unwelcome guest at a peripheral lesion of her own making. If the guest be one simple innocuous thing or substance, then as soon as that is detruded the matter is ended the abscess heals.

If the surgeon lances, in such a case, this aid to Nature would under circumstances be rational and sensible. If the stasis itself be the whole affair, then Kellgrenism would be right to disperse, for then an outlet would not be needed, since there would be nothing to let out. In this stasis-abscess, gentle pressive coaxing aid would be the most rational, the 'free incision' merely a woodhacker's mode of doing the same thing. i.e., getting rid of the stagnation.

But the pre-fistular abscess differs widely from the two kinds of abscess just mentioned. It is not a stasis-abscess, for its stasis is a means to an end, the mean being to mortify a bit of tissue to form an outlet; and the end being the detrusion of not a simple innocuous thing or substance, but some *organismic morbid product* that is being daily and hourly produced, and therefore needs daily and hourly discharge, in fact a constantly open issue, which a fistula in my opinion often is. If I am correct in this view, it must follow that a fistula should not be made to heal up by any and every local means but the fistula patient should be cured by internal constitutional treatment.

I find myself quite unable to believe that causing the fistula to heal up is in any sense a real cure; on the contrary, I believe this proceeding to be bad practice, and very harmful in its consequences for the future health and well-being of the patients. Neither am I able to conceive how any kind of treatment by manipulation could possibly alter the state of one's constitution: a syphilitic, a strumous, a sycotic, a psoric individual would so far as I can see, be just as syphilitic as strumous, as sycotic, as psoric after being manipulated as before.

## CONCLUSION

Having now, as I submit practically demonstrated the feasibility of a radical, cure of fistula by medicines, I claim for this method of cure in the aggregate superiority over all others superior in the following particulars:

1. It is radical, in that the remedies can be chosen so that the internal causes of the fistular process are attacked and overcome.

2. It is painless.

3. It does not interfere with the mode of life or occupation of the sufferers.

4. There are no ill after-effects to the nervous system from shock, such as may, and often do follow operations.

5.  It is safe in that the chest and other affections are ameliorated *pari passu* with the general cure of the constitutional crisis.

6.  It is effective in those cases in which surgery fails because the fistula will not heal.

7.  It is philosophic, being consonant with the true wisdom of self-preservation.

8.  It is scientific, the remedies being chosen in accordance with the data of pharmacology derived from positive experiments on the healthy.

    'Now! I can go no further; well or ill, it is done'

# PART II

Since the First Edition of this small work on the medicinal cure of fistula went to press a considerable number of cases of fistula of various kinds have passed under my professional care, so that I can now raise my voice with a little greater authority, and maintain more strongly than ever that the treatment of the fistular disease by operation and locally healing measures is irrational and harmful. True it is that some cases of fistula are very difficult to cure, particularly where the number of fistula in one individual is very great. I once counted eighteen in one person and these cases that have existed for many years and in which the lining of the fistula has become dense and hard, and constantly accustomed to secrete almost like the lining membrane of a cyst. Still even here a cure–a perfect cure can be effected if the physician will take the trouble and the sufferers will have the patience.

It frequently happens that the fistula is only one of the ailments of a given patient, and not always the most important either. This must be well considered. It might not unreasonably be asked of me, what, then is the fistular disease if the fistula proper be not the malady? Well, I find that a considerable number of constitutional taints run out through fistulas, and I hope, with time, to give direct information on this important subject, out at present I must be content to narrate a few cases of cure, from which my readers will be able to draw certain conclusions themselves.

Perhaps by the time a third edition comes round I may be able to give a classification of fistulas according to their pathologic qualities deduced partly from their genealogies and partly from the known actions of the remedies that have proved curative of them. Certainly there are liver-fistulas, i.e. fistulas of hepatic origin, and here the liver must be cured or the fistulas cannot be. Certainly there are lung-fistulas i.e., fistulas of pulmonary origin. Here the lungs must be first cured, or the sequal brings constitutional retribution; here we must be especially aware of operations, for if this kind of fistula be forcibly closed, phthisis comes anon.

Certainly there are spleen fistulas, or fistulas of splenic origin. I will give presently a striking example of a splenic fistula. But this part of my subject is new, and needs much thinking about before going further, so I will simply proceed to the narration of a few, instructive cases of cure of fistula by medicines.

## CASE OF HEREDITARY FISTULA

The gentleman whose case is first narrated in this book sent me a friend of his suffering from fistula, as does also this latter's father. This friend came to me on November 2, 1891, telling me that he had a perineal abscess, which broke six weeks ago and left a fistula which at date is again gathering. He early seeks advice, because of his father's chronic condition. Patient has, besides a chronic winter cough, very hard; otherwise he is in excellent condition, a trifle stout, perhaps. There are no indurated glands anywhere to be found, but he gets a little acne here and there. He suffers a good deal of pain during defecation.

In December, 1892 the fistula had quite disappeared and has not since returned, though I think it very probable that he may have a few more flickerings here and there yet, though of course he may not.

The chief remedies were *Bacillinum, Thuja occidentalis, Sabina, Levico aqua, Hydrasitis canadensis, Hepar sulphur, Acidum nitricum.* There were numerous gatherings of pus before the cure was accomplished.

## CASE OF FISTULA CURED BY URTICA URENS

According to my views almost every fistula has a cause more or less remote from the fistula proper; we might almost compare the fistula to the crater of a volcano.

Where a given organ seems to be the starting point of the cause of a fistula, an appropriate remedy of that organ will at times aid much in its cure. I will now relate a case which appears to have been cured by one organ-remedy alone, viz., by the notable spleen remedy *Urtica urens.* The discovery that *Urtica urens* has a specific influence on the spleen, I claim as my own.

An unmarried gentleman came to consult me for fistula just before Christmas, 1890.

Originally there appears to have been a fall, and then an abscess. Patient was operated upon for his fistula in 1886, and again in 1887, but without avail. He was in fairly good health all the time, and though he still had his fistula when he came to me, notwithstanding the two operations, he did not come because he was ill, but because he was desirous of getting married. He complained only of one thing, viz. he was always very chilly.

I examined him with very great care, and apart from the fistula itself I could find nothing wrong with him except that he had a very greatly hypertrophied spleen.

About two ounces of *Urtica urens* spread over a number of weeks, seemingly cured him for he reported himsef as cured in the early summer of 1891. In July of that year he went up the river, and reported some swelling of the old fistular region. The *Urtica urens* was repeated, and, I believe, cured him: I am not quite sure but he had previously reported himself cure, then he reported the swelling and a few weeks later he got married. I think he must be cured because he passes my door about twice a month to see a mutual friend of us both, and this mutual friend is in the habit of referring to this cure of fistula by medicines. Still I have not examined him, and thus do not vouch for its being a complete cure. I regard it as a fistula of splenic origin. and hence the fistula would heal as soon as the spleen was cured.

## POST MALARIAL FISTULA IN THE BACK

The following case of fistula is unique in my experience, and not far from being absolutely, unique in the annals of fistulae.

In the fall of the year 1890 a gentleman brought his wife to me; they had just returned from India. In June 1890, the lady, had a fall in Bombay, whereupon she miscarried and before she could recover she developed malarial fever. Then abscess formed in the womb and also in the back, about the region corresponding to the part lying between the left-hand end of the pancreas and the lower part of the spleen. On inspection I found a freely discharging fistula, with much inflammation around it, occupying the first described region of the back. The spleen was very much enlarged. Patient is a large woman, 30 years old of age, very bloodless and washed out looking, and very ill in herself. As I find that *Urtica urens* has a strong affinity for the spleen, I thought I would just bring that organ back to the normal therewith (which I have very often done before). I gave her twenty drops of the *Urtica urens* tincture daily. This was on September 12, 1890.

October 6-A very great change for the better has taken place in the patient; the spleen has gone down, the circumfistular inflammation has greatly diminished, and patient looks and feels much better. The medicine to be continued in a smaller dose.

October 20 - Patient continues to improve.

The fistula has closed; a little throat cough. seemingly from a cold.

R

*Phosphorus* 3 and *Chelidonium majus* θ.

November 19 - The fistula has healed up patient has had her second period since the miscarriage, and there was very much uterine pain at the time. There has been a slight attack of malarial fever with night sweats.

*Helianthus annus* θ six drops in water night and morning.

December 10-Menses normal; a lump flat of the size of a baby's open hand has come in the left breast. Regarding this as from the uterus, I gave *Bursa pastoris* 1x six drops night and morning.

January 7, 1891-Breast normal; some pain in the liver; much less pain at the last period; a bit of a cough.

R

*Carduus marianus*, five drops night and morning.

February 6-One bad bout of fever, and since then very well. The fistula remains perfectly healed. I heard from the husband a good while subsequently, telling me there had been no relapse.

## FISTULA PROCTALGIA-GRAVE DEPRESSION OF SPIRITS

A city merchant, about 50 years of age, came to me in the month of March 1890, in very great distress of mind on account of his fistula or rather, on account of the fact that three different surgeons-one an eminent specialist for diseases of the rectum had declared an operation imperative. The idea of being operated upon had almost unhinged his mind, and he was seemingly neglecting an important business; he could talk of nothing but his fistula and the impending operation. The fistula was very small very painful, and had made his life miserable for about three months. During the past six weeks he has lost 16 pounds in weight. The proctalgia he described as 'terrible, day and night'. At first *Hydrastis canadensis* took the pain away, and it returned; *Variolinum C.* I thought indicated, but it did no good. *Hydrastis canadensis* was again resorted to, but it did not help, and patient literally ran about wildly from the pain, often standing with legs apart with much bearing down.

On April 23, my note runs thus: 'No amelioration. The tongue is gouty; he compares the pain to that caused by nettles. His sufferings are awful.'

℞

*Tc Urtica urens* 1x, ten drops in water every four hours.

May 9 - These drops cured the burning pain in three days.

℞

*Phytolaccinum* 3x

June 4 - No return of the pain at all.

Patient has regained much of his lost weight and is now as hilarious as he was previously depressed. At the seat there is nothing observable save a flap of flesh at the side of the anal mouth.

℞

*Sodium silicatum* θ.

July 2 - Not happy at the seat; mentally apprehensive; a close inspection shows, hidden behind the before

named flap of flesh, a small wart with a bleeding fissure
athwart it.

℞

*Sambucus nigra* θ.

Patient was discharged quite cured and in
fine physical and mental condition just fourteen
months from the beginning of his treatment. During
the remaining part of his treatment he received
from me *Chelidonium majus* θ, *Urtica urens*, in
several differing strengths. *Hecla lava 30, Kalium
iodatum 30, Calcarea carbonicum* C. C., and finally
*Silicea terra* C.

In this case I did use one local application, viz.,
powdered *Thuja occidentalis* applied direct to the
bleeding comb like processes behind the fleshy flap,
and of this flap its shrivelled remains are still *in situ*.

## FISTULA-VERRUCOUS GROWTH AND HAEMORRHOIDS

Early in the year 1890 a gentleman verging on 70 years
of age came from the country to consult me for anal
trouble characterized by a sticky, gummy discharge. An
examination of the part disclosed a wart-like growth of
the size of a walnut, and also a pile. I could not find any

fistula. A month later I found the mouth of the fistula leading into a funnel shaped discharging cavity.

He remained under treatment for a year during which time the fistula healed and patient greatly improved in health. *Bacillinum* C., *Hydrastis canadensis*, θ, *Phytolaccinum* 3x, *Sodium silicatum*, *Sambucus nigra* θ, were the chief remedies. The growth was much smaller when patient discharged himself, and was wishful to continue the treatment longer, but he was comfortable in himself, the anal region being dry since the fistula healed up. His digestion so very much improved that he would not be bothered with any more physicking.

## CASE OF FISTULA IN A LADY

A married lady, 33 years of age, was brought to me by her husband in the spring of 1891 to be treated for fistula-in-ano, that had been a source of annoyance and trouble for a little over two years, seemingly starting from the retention of a dead foetus at that period, which was then thought to have been three weeks dead. At a previous confinement there had been considerable laceration of the perineum, the sequel of which had had to be remedied by the electrocautery, and thus a somewhat imperfect closing of the sphincter ani has come about, and loose stools being the rule, the poor lady had a sad time of it. A fistula alone is a humiliating possession but when faecal incontinence is added, the condition becomes fearful. The fistula was situated at the back, and was in the habit of closing for a few days, and then it would burst and discharge. Besides the fistula and an inadequate sphincter muscle, there were piles that however, did not cause very much inconvenience. Patient was put upon *Thuja occidentalis* 30 in infrequent doses for one month.

The case was seen from month to month, and required some pretty careful differential drug diagnosis before it was permanently cured, patient being discharged quite well in the month of July 1892. The chief remedies used were *Bacillinum M.* and CC. given altogether during four separate months. *Helianthus annuus* θ, *Bursa pastoris* θ, *Kalium iodatum.* 3 trit. and 30, and *Bovista lycoperdon* 3 trit., have come into play in between as indicated. In this case I was guided to the use of the remedies from the state of the cervical glands and the circumscribed flush of the cheeks, and by the patient's various symptoms.

# CASE Of PREFISTULAR CELLULITIS DISPERSED

Sometimes one is fortunate enough to get cases of prefistular gathering soon enough to prevent both abscess and fistula. Thus a middle-aged merchant from the Midlands came under my care in the fall of 1891, with a lump at the seat that was giving rise to inconvenience and anxiety to the patient, partly because he was quite familiar with fistula in his own family. He was well in three months; during the first half of the time he was taking *Arnica montana* 1, twenty drops a day in water. This took away much of the swelling and nearly all the hardening and then I gave *Chelidonium majus* $\theta$ on organopathic lines.

That we here prevented both abscess and fistula hardly admits of any doubt.

# CASE OF RECTAL ABSCESSES AND FISTULA

In the month of January, 1892, a London professional man came under my care. Two months previously he had had a very large abscess of the rectum, which had been freely incised but would not heal, and a fistular state remained, with much discharge; or, rather, I should say that there remained a hole in the flesh fully two inches long, discharging matter profusely.

And notwithstanding the profuse discharge from this gash, there was another large gathering on the other side of the anus which the surgeon was on the point of operating on.

Patient's father and one of his sisters had died of phthisis. I began the treatment with *Ignatia amara* 1, alternated with *Hydrastis Canadensis* θ, because of patient's low nervous anorexic condition. This was continued for a fortnight, much to his comfort and feeling of well being, when early in February gout broke out in his right foot. This was met with *Aconitum napellus* 6 and *Bryonia alba* θ. With the outbreak of the gout the activity at the seat lessened, and the gash in the flesh began to heal from the bottom. I had applied nothing to the wound, but rather encouraged its activity.

The treatment was continued–patient all the while attending to his professional duties with some ups and downs, till May 25, 1893, when patient was discharged cured, and in capital health and spirits. Many remedies were needed and used, and of these the chief were: *Bacillinum* C.C. and C.; *Bryonia alba* θ; *Bellis perennis* θ; *Chelidonium majus* θ; *Chionanthus virginicus* θ; *Natrium muriaticum*; 6 trit.; *Levico aqua* (strong); *Thuja occidentalis* 30 and *Lycopodium clavatum* 6.

To give the reasons for giving the various medicines would occupy more space than I can here afford, but there were three leading ideas underlying them viz.:

1. The hereditary phthisic taint.

2. The enlarged unhealthy liver.

3. The gout, and then we had to meet –

   a. The debility

   b. The anaemia

   c. The anorexia

   d. The neurasthenia, the last-named being a potent factor in the sum; at any rate, neurasthenia cannot be operated away.

## GRAVE CASE OF RECTO-VAGINAL FISTULA

A childless lady, many years married, 42 years of age, came to consult me for recto-vaginal fistula early in the year 1890. Both of her parents died about 80 years of age in fact her mother lived to be 82; and all her brothers and sisters being still alive and well and patient herself being of very fine build. I was quite astonished to hear the following narration of her health-history and present state:- Formerly had a fearful cough, remaining as a sequel of a pneumonia, the cough, being so bad that some thought it from a form of asthma. Formerly very thin then stout (large, not obese), i.e., polysarcous and now losing flesh. It is noteworthy that when she began to get perineal abscesses her cough entirely disappeared.

In childhood she had had measles, whooping-cough and scarlatina in the proper way, since then a carbuncle on her right arm. Menses copious; she is weary and tired; tongue gouty, with no 'strawberry' pips (a very important point); considerable leucorrhoea; she is very chilly. Notwithstanding the history of pneumonia, and notwithstanding the very bad cough that disappeared as soon as the prefistular abscesses began to appear, I still could not regard the fistula as in any sense indicative of a phthisic taint, but I came to the conclusion that it was a case of genuine vaccinosic manifestations; the chilliness, the leucorrhoea, the polysarcia, the pithy tongue, the sterility all, in my judgement, pointing at any rate to the hydrogenoid constitution of Grauvogle.

The fistula was sequential to abscesses at the spot, and patient stated that it had gathered twelve times.

Patient had been operated on by a distinguished surgeon three months previously but without success, and further and very much more serious operation was in prospect, and hence the lady's visit to me. Now it happened that this lady's house was, and is, the rendez-vous of quite a number of medical men all sincerely attached to this lady's husband. 'Nearly all our friends happen to be medical men', said she, 'and my husband has discussed the question of the possibility of my fistula being cured with medicines, and they all declare it to be absolutely impossible, and my husband is so sure that it is impossible that he has refused to come with me'.

Still in an aside she gave me to understand that he privately hoped she would come, on the off-chance of a cure, and so avoid the alarmingly radical operation in contemplation.

It is to be remembered that an operation for fistula depends a good deal on the kind of person to be operated upon as well as its position. In this case the position was most awkward, and the quantity of tissue through which the incisions would have to be made very considerable.

In the left groin gland are indurated and enlarged moreover, they become tender just before each gathering and remain so till it has burst and discharged.

In as much as many medical men had declared this case absolutely unamenable medicinal treatment, and two of them watched the progress of the case, in as much as one operation had already failed it was performed in a well-known hospital, it being considered too considerable to be conveniently done at home and in as much as my diagnosis will be unacceptable to almost all medical men even to many of my best friends and colleagues, I am going to enter into very full details of the cases, to motive my diagnosis and the line of treatment such diagnosis compelled.

If any of my readers takes an interest in the question of the constitutional effects of the poison of vaccination, I refer such a one to my little treatise on the subject, entitled '*Vaccinosis and its Cure by Thuja*'.

In this case patient had been vaccinated four times. From this fact, and for the reasons already given (symptoms negative and positive). I considered I had to do with a genuine and severe case of vaccinosis.

I began the treatment on January 10,1890, with the matrix tincture of *Hydrastis cananadensis* giving eight drops in water three times a day.

February 3-The leucorrhoea is not so bad; the place is angry, but the swelling is less. Patient feels better. 'I am picking up'. Feels very cold always, and she is also cold to the touch. Sleeps lightly, and gets the fidgets in her legs.

R

*Thuja occidentalis* 30, infrequently.

February 17-Markedly better; no trouble with the gathering whatever; no discharge from the fistula worth while; no menses for six weeks; still feels very chilly; parts no longer swollen, no tenderness of inguinal glands; much better of the tiredness and weariness.

No medicine, to allow the remedial action already set up to continue undisturbedly.

March 7-No pain, and no gathering; one scanty menstruation; she is always cold; the enlargement of the inguinal glands has disappeared; not so tired or weary.

R

*Vaccininum* C; very infrequently.

March 26-No gathering; not so cold; leucorrhoea better; has a cold, with a little cough; is gaining flesh.

R

*Ceanothus americanus*, ten drops in water night and morning.

April 12-No gathering; feels less cold; and the left hypochondrium is less uneasy.

R

*Hydrastis canadensis* as before, but in a smaller dose.

May 22-Menses set in three weeks ago, and still continue; left ovary is tender.

℞

*Juniperus sabina* 30, very infrequently.

June 30 - Fistula quite gone, and almost well in herself.

℞

*Cupressus lawsoniana* 30, very infrequently.

I heard no more of the patient till the following November, when she came, telling me she had continued quite well, but the last week or so she had felt slight tenderness where the fistula used to be and it seemed as if it might gather.

℞

*Thuja occidentalis* 30, as before.

February 9, 1891-Has been quite well but the old fistula is again active and gathering.

℞

*Silicea terra* 30, ten drops every three hours.

This was followed by complete cure and capital health till.

July 13-When patient again called, telling me she felt as if it were going to gather again, but objectively there was absolutely nothing abnormal.

R

*Thuja occidentalis* 30, as before.

At this point I ceased keeping notes of the case, although patient called to see me on two or three occasions for little threatenings and flickerings, but these have now long ceased.

On May 19, 1893, patient told me that, she had been quite well in all respects for nine months, and she was in blooming health.

In this case I made the diagnosis of vaccinosis and base the treatment thereon. As soon as the blood disease was much lessened the fistula healed up, and as soon as the blood disease was quite cured the flickerings in the old fistula ceased entirely. The healing process shows itself also in this case, as in so many others, as gentle, gradual and with candle-like flickerings until the disease becomes quite extinguished.

Could any more conclusive proof be given of the constitutional nature of fistula?

I used no local measures whatever.

# INDEX

5

2